CW00395178

pilates

pilates

101 energizing exercises

Yvonne Worth

MQP

Caution
If you are pregnant, or suffer from any illness or injury,
you should seek medical advice before beginning any
exercise program.

This book is intended as an informational guide only
and is not to be used as a substitute for professional
medical care or treatment. Neither the author nor the
publisher can be held responsible for any damage,
injury, or otherwise resulting from the use of the
information in this book.

Published by MQ Publications Limited
12 The Ivories,
6-8 Northampton Street
London N1 2HY
Tel: 020 7359 2244
Fax: 020 7359 1616
email: mail@mqpublications.com
website: www.mqpublications.com

Copyright © MQ Publications 2004
Text copyright © Yvonne Worth 2004

Series Editor: Karen Ball, MQ Publications
Editorial Director: Ljiljana Baird, MQ Publications
Senior Designer: Victoria Bevan, MQ Publications
Photography by Mike Prior
Design by Balley Design Associates

All rights reserved. No part of this publication may
be reproduced or transmitted in any form or by any
means, electronic or mechanical, including photocopy,
recording, or any information storage and retrieval
system now known or to be invented without
permission in writing from the publishers.

ISBN 1-84072-586-9

Printed in France by *Partenaires-Livres*® (JL)

1 3 5 7 9 0 8 6 4 2

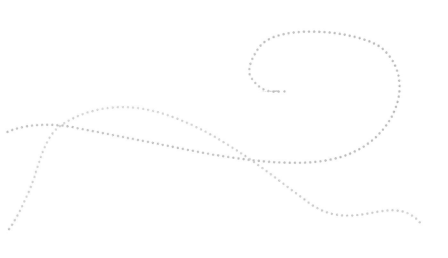

contents

Introduction

Given the hectic nature of modern-day living and the pressures that we constantly find ourselves under, it's hardly surprising for all of us—even the fittest, healthiest, most dynamic among us—to find our energy levels flagging a little from time to time and ourselves in need of a little help to get us through the day.

The Pilates system of exercise provides the perfect antidote to a demanding schedule, offering a system of gentle, effective movements that reduce tension; counteract the effects of stress; improve breathing, posture, and alignment; develop muscle tone; increase flexibility, and restore vitality.

Drawing its inspiration from the Pilates method, this book contains tips that will help you put a spring back in your step, clear your mind, and give you the vitality boost you need—in body, mind, and spirit.

Whether you're simply looking for the occasional pick-me-up, or to make more radical changes to your daily routine, this book is packed with invaluable suggestions on how to make those improvements and enhance your life.

Key benefits of Pilates

- Develops core abdominal strength.
- Helps you develop a leaner body by lengthening and stretching muscles.
- Improves balance, poise, stability, and flexibility.
- It is suitable for anyone, regardless of age or level of fitness.

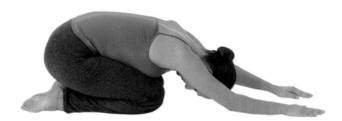

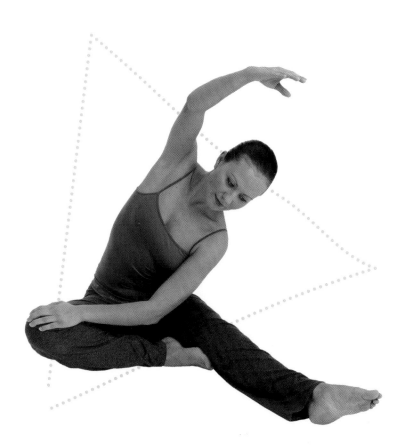

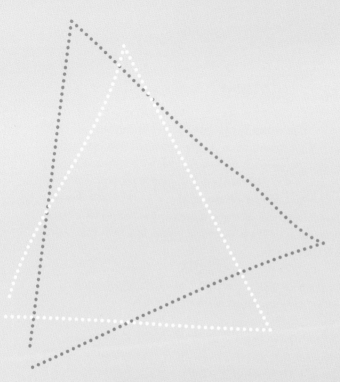

Back to basics

Simple ways to improve your
energy levels throughout the day.

1 Correct posture

Good posture is essential to our general well-being and our ability to function efficiently and think clearly. Too frequently we forget about our posture, allowing ourselves to sit for hours in discomfort, and then wonder why we feel tired, stiff, and achy, and unable to function properly. Taking a minute or two at least once a day to correct your posture will give you a moment or two to focus your energy back into your body, clear your mind, and help you feel on top of the world.

❶ Stand with your feet in parallel, hip-width apart, arms resting gently by your sides. Breath normally.

❷ Focus your attention on your feet, checking that your weight is evenly distributed. Now bring your attention up to your knees and make sure they are "soft" (slightly bent).

❸ Relax your shoulders, allowing them to drop down away from your ears, but without forcing them back or rounding them forward. Now bring your attention to your spine. Lengthen up through your spine and neck picturing a thread running through your spinal cord, dropping down through your tailbone to the floor and up and out of the top of your head to the ceiling.

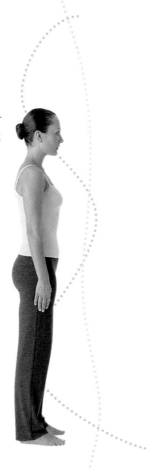

2 Breathing

❶ Stand or sit comfortably with your feet in parallel, hip-width apart. Keeping your shoulders dropped and your spine lengthened, place your hands at the base of your ribs, with your middle fingers touching.

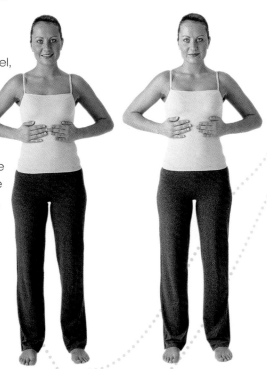

❷ Keeping the upper part of the chest relaxed, inhale through your nose, imagining that the breath is being drawn into the lower part of your lungs, expanding your rib cage outwards and pulling your fingertips away from each other. Exhale through your mouth and release. Repeat several times, but avoid hyperventilating.

Try this same exercise lying on your back in semi-supine (with your knees raised and your feet in parallel, hip-width apart). As you inhale feel the back of your rib cage expanding as it presses into the floor.

3 Fresh Air

For an extra boost of energy, take in some fresh air at least once a day—if it is not possible to practice your breathing exercises (or even your regular daily workout) outdoors or by an open window, take a short, brisk walk each day in the open air (in a traffic-free zone, naturally).

4 Centering

In Pilates the "core," or "center," or "powerhouse" is extremely important. This is located at the body's natural center of gravity and is approximately 2in (6cm) below the navel. Pilates moves are performed using the contraction of the abdominal muscles (the central core). Working from this center allows us to build strength and stamina, lengthening and stretching the body without any risk of strain or injury. Activating the abdominals is a simple movement that can be done at any time and only takes a few seconds, but will quickly improve your core strength and enhance your feeling of well-being.

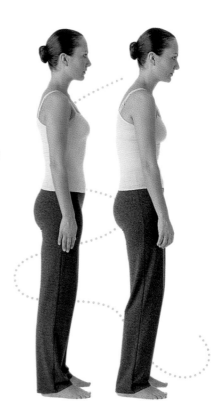

❶ In either a sitting or standing position, contract the abdominal muscles, drawing the navel back toward the spine while, at the same time, pulling up on the pelvic floor muscle (as if interrupting the flow of urine).

❷ Avoid flattening out the lumbar spine and rounding the shoulders as you do this.

5 Think positive

The controlled, flowing Pilates movements can improve gland and organ function, enhancing your general health as well as boosting energy: as you exercise, clear your mind of any negative thoughts, allowing positive, uplifting energy to flow through your mind and body.

6 Sitting and standing with ease

❶ Sit on the edge of a chair with your feet flat on the floor. Tilt your pelvis forward, flattening out your back slightly.

❷ Now reverse the movement tilting your pelvis back and arching very slightly forward.

❸ Keep moving gently between these two points until you find the mid-point where you are comfortably positioned with a slight natural curve in your lower back—this is your "neutral."

❹ Try finding neutral while standing, keeping your knees soft. Avoid rounding your shoulders or flattening out your lower back.

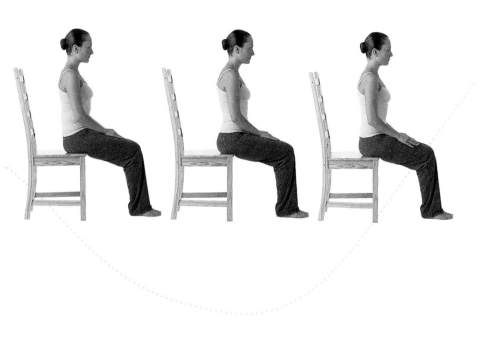

7 Body balance

This exercise is excellent as an initial warm-up, or can be used throughout the day as a quick pick-me-up and gentle stretch.

❶ Stand with your feet in parallel, hip-width apart. Check that your knees are soft, your arms relaxed and your shoulders dropped down away from your ears. Focus your eyes directly in front of you and inhale.

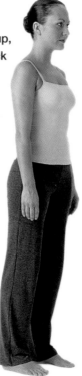

❷ Contract your abdominals, drawing your navel toward your spine, then exhale and allow your heels to raise up gently away from the ground. As you lift, keeping the movement smooth and controlled, focus your eyes on a point straight in front of you and lengthen up through the spine and neck, imagining the crown of the head lifting straight up toward the ceiling and the tailbone releasing down to the floor.

❸ Keep exhaling as you roll up onto your toes (avoid dropping your ankles out to the sides as you do this), then inhale, contract your abdominals and exhale as you roll your feet softly back down to the floor, keeping as much length in your spine as possible. Repeat 5–10 times.

8 Fitness and diet

To function efficiently and effectively we need to take the time and make the effort to look after ourselves properly. Regular exercise, a healthy diet, sufficient rest, reduced stress, and a positive attitude to life are all key elements in our general well-being. Fortunately, even small changes to our lifestyle can have a profound effect, boosting vitality and improving our levels of energy, both physically and mentally. Getting fit need not require hours spent at the gym each week—simply setting aside a few minutes a day to do a few simple stretches will quickly show positive results—both in the way you feel and the way you look: improved quality of sleep, increased vitality, improved flexibility and stamina, increased circulation leading to clearer skin and brighter eyes, reduced tension, and elimination of aches and pains.

9 Cardio vascular exercise

Alongside any Pilates regime, you are recommended to include some form of cardiovascular exercise each week—to raise your heart rate, and improve your circulation. You do not need to sign up for aerobics classes though; a brisk walk, a swim, or even running up and down stairs a few times will be equally effective.

10 Water, water

Sipping a little water at various times throughout the day can give an immediate boost to your flagging energy levels, ensuring that your mechanism avoids risk of dehydration and toxins are flushed efficiently from your body. Resist the temptation to reach for a caffeine or sugar hit when you feel in need of a break—this may give you an instant fix, but it will be shortlived, leaving you even more depleted. Instead, drink a glass of water or a cup of herb tea and take the time to do a few stretches to stimulate your circulation and restore your energy. Always drink water after exercising, to replace any that you may lose as you work out.

11 Neutral position

"Neutral spine" or "neutral" is an essential aspect of Pilates and is based upon the natural position for the spine. Maintaining the natural contours of the spine as we work, rather than forcing the body into unnatural and uncomfortable positions, and acquiring the habit of keeping the spine in this position, improves our posture and balance and reduces risk of strain or injury as we go about our daily activities. Lying on your back in neutral (with your knees raised and a slight gap under your waist) and focusing on your breath will refresh and recharge you.

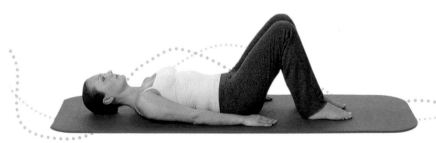

12 Side bend

Sit in a comfortable upright position, hands on your thighs or knees, palms upward. Close your eyes and start to pay attention to your breathing.

❶ Sit on the floor with your left leg extended, and rest your right foot against the inner thigh. Inhale, taking your arms out to the sides at shoulder level.

❷ Contract your abdominals and exhale, curving your body over toward your left knee. As you stretch, take your left hand onto your right knee and curve your arm and hand up and over your head, creating a stretch along the right side of the body. Inhale and return to center. Repeat 3–5 times, then switch position and repeat on the other side.

13 Rest and relaxation

To keep your energy levels at their optimum it is essential that you make sure you get sufficient rest. Try to get a good night's sleep, but also find times throughout the day to unwind and let go of any tension or worries, as these will quickly drain you. Even a ten-minute cat-nap will help revive you and restore your energy, while making the effort to engage in physical activity, instead of spending the evening curled up in front of the television, will refresh and invigorate you.

14 Quick energy releaser

Taking a deep breath and checking your posture (returning to "neutral") at various times throughout the day can be a great energy-releaser, freeing up any energy wasted on sitting or standing uncomfortably.

15 One-leg circles (side)

❶ Lie on your left side with your left knee bent up toward your body, your right leg extended. Stretch your arms out above your head, grasping your right wrist with your left hand and resting your head on your arm. Inhale.

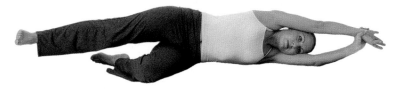

❷ Contract the abdominals and raise your left leg to hip level. Exhale and, lengthening the leg as you stretch, draw 5 small circles with the right foot in one direction and 5 times in the opposite direction. Repeat 3 times, then change position and repeat for the other side.

16 Prayer pose

❶ Kneel on all fours, with your knees directly below your hips and your hands below your shoulders.

❷ Gently lower your body until you are sitting back on your heels with your arms stretched out in front of

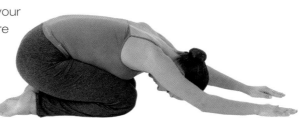

you, fingers forward. Keeping the spine lengthened and the shoulders relaxed, drop your forehead down toward the floor. Hold this position for 5–10 breaths, longer if you prefer, using each out breath to let go of a little more tension.

Variation: Try this exercise using this alternative arm position: as you lower your body, allow your arms to slide back either side of your legs, with the palms facing upward.

17 Quick-fix breathing

For times when you feel your energy start to flag, give yourself an immediate boost by taking 3 deep breaths (in through the nose and out through the mouth), allowing the breath to clear your head and calm your thoughts: as you exhale, imagine that you are letting go of all tension, worry, and fatigue, leaving you feeling fresh and relaxed.

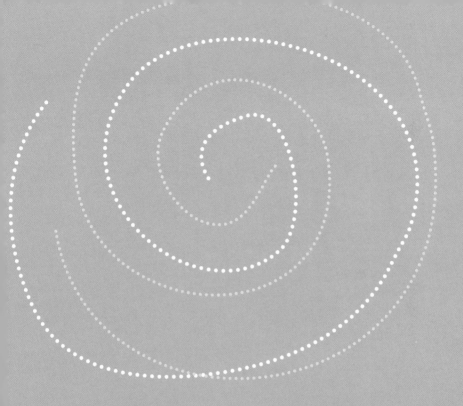

Getting physical

Hints on hitting peak form and
staying there.

18 Arm swings

❶ Stand with your feet in parallel, hip-width apart, knees soft. Inhale and raise your arms toward the ceiling, keeping your shoulders dropped and your arms and hands relaxed.

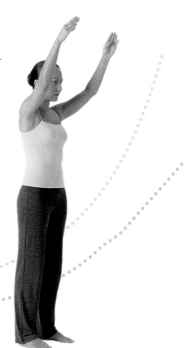

❷ Contract the abdominals and exhale, swinging your arms down toward the floor and back behind you slightly in a slow smooth gesture, allowing your knees to bend and your head and spine to curve over as you swing.

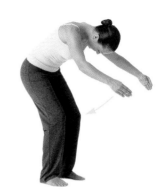

❸ Inhale as you continue the move swinging your arms forward and gently rolling back up to the starting position. Repeat 5–10 times.

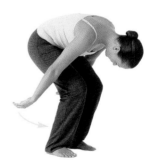

19 Push up

❶ Stand in neutral with your feet hip-width apart. Inhale, contract your abdominals, then exhale, dropping your head forward, and rolling down through the spine, one vertebra at a time. Keep your knees soft and your arms relaxed.

❷ When you have rolled as far as you can, bend your knees and ease your hands onto the floor. Inhale, contract the abdominals and exhale, walking your hands slowly forward and dropping onto your knees.

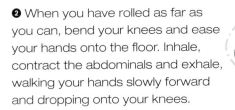

❸ Inhale, and then exhale as you lower your upper body down to the floor then inhale as you raise it back again, keeping your hips level. Repeat 5–10 times, exhaling as you lower and inhaling as you raise up.

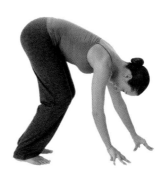

❹ Exhale and walk your hands back, taking your weight onto your feet, then rolling up through the spine to standing.

20 Neck pull prep

❶ Sit on the floor with your feet together, knees raised, and your spine and neck lengthened. Inhale, contract the abdominals and exhale, tucking the tailbone under slightly and slowly curling down through the spine.

❷ Keep rolling back until you start to feel some resistance in the abdominals, then inhale and allow your left arm to float upward, keeping your shoulders dropped. Exhale and release the arm as you roll slowly back to center. Repeat 5–10 times, using alternate arms.

21 Waking up and getting going

Start the day on a positive note by having a good stretch. As you tumble out of bed, stand with your feet slightly apart, lift your arms to the ceiling and stretch as far as you can, raising yourself up onto your toes and reaching out through your fingertips. As you stretch, make yourself yawn—as loudly as possible—and blink your eyes several times.

22 Early-morning energy booster

To kickstart your day, squeeze the juice of half a lemon into a mug of hot water (and sweeten with a little honey, if necessary) and sip slowly. This is a great way to boost your system and will leave you feeling energized and prepared for anything.

23 Putting a spring in your step

Getting into a routine of regular exercise is an excellent way to put a spring in your step and keep your energy flowing throughout the day. Adding a few minutes of stretching into your morning routine will quickly enhance your feeling of well-being and improve your levels of fitness and flexibility.

24 Healthy breakfast

Breakfast is the most important meal of the day—it is essential to eat good, nourishing food before you launch yourself into your day. Fruit, muesli, and yogurt are excellent breakfast foods and if you're someone who really needs a hit of coffee, this is the time for it, as you have the rest of the day to get it out of your system.

25 One-leg circles

Lie on the floor in the neutral position. Float your left leg up until your knee is at a right angle, with the shin parallel to the floor. Place the fingers of your right hand on your right knee and, as you exhale, draw 5–10 small circles with your knee in one direction, then 5–10 circles in the opposite direction, pausing to inhale as you change direction. Repeat for the other leg. Repeat the sequence 3–5 times in total.

Variation—intermediate/advanced

For a more challenging exercise, extend the leg and rest your arms at your sides. As you circle, keep lengthening the leg out of the hip, making sure that the opposite leg remains still, with the knee pointing straight up to the ceiling.

26 One-leg kick

❶ Lie face down with your arms placed close to the body, elbows in line with your shoulders, your palms resting on the floor. Contract the abdominals and exhale, stretching gently up through your chest, lengthening along the spine and back of the neck.

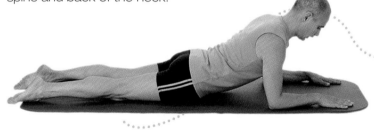

❷ Bend your right knee, bringing your foot up toward the ceiling, but keeping your thigh in contact with the floor. Inhale, contract the abdominals and exhale, kicking the right heel toward the right buttock. Kick again, then inhale and lower as you bend the left knee and raise the left foot. Repeat 5–10 times on each side.

❸ For a more challenging variation, raise your hips off the ground and extend the right leg, raising it to just below hip level.

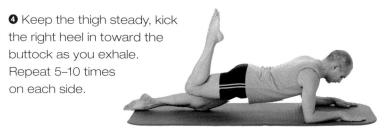

❹ Keep the thigh steady, kick the right heel in toward the buttock as you exhale. Repeat 5–10 times on each side.

27 Put your best foot forward

Our feet support us throughout our waking life and yet they are a part of the body that we tend to neglect. Giving your feet a five-minute massage will make your toes twinkle and leave you feeling grounded and energized.

28 Hip twist

❶ Sit with your legs extended out in front of you, ankles and knees together. Place your hands on the floor slightly behind your hips, fingertips lightly touching the floor. Inhale, raising your legs, leaning back and balancing yourself with your fingertips.

❷ Exhale, contract the abdominals and curve your legs upward and over to the left, then down and around to draw a circle with your feet.

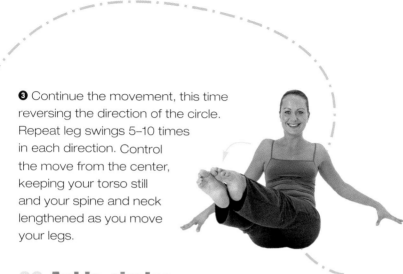

❸ Continue the movement, this time reversing the direction of the circle. Repeat leg swings 5–10 times in each direction. Control the move from the center, keeping your torso still and your spine and neck lengthened as you move your legs.

29 Ankle circles

❶ Either lie on your back with your knees raised, or sit up, if you prefer. Lift one leg and, supporting the thigh with your hands, slowly circle the ankle outward 10 times then reverse the direction and circle inward 10 times.

❷ Change legs and repeat for the other side.

30 Breaktime boosters

Always take short, regular breaks throughout the day. If you tend to be stuck in one position (e.g. at your desk) for hours it is vital that you take "time out." A good time to stop and recharge can be at "natural" breaks such as the end of a telephone call, or when you have completed a task. Alternatively, set an alarm every hour to remind you to stop and recharge—drink a little water, take a few deep breaths, and do some stretching (or run up and down a flight of stairs.)

31 Eye cupping

Air conditioning and computer screens can quickly tire the eyes. For a quick eye-refresher, rub your hands together several times to warm the palms, rest your elbows on a hard surface, close your eyes and cup your palms over them for a minute or two.

32 Standing pecs stretch

❶ Stand with your feet in parallel, hip-width apart, arms behind your back at waist level, hands together. Inhale, contract the abdominals and lengthen the spine.

❷ Exhale and slowly take your hands down behind you, drawing your shoulder blades down and back. Repeat 5 times.

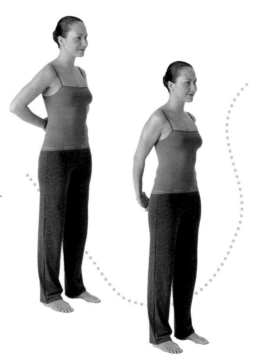

33 Rolling down

❶ Stand with your feet in parallel, hip-width apart, arms resting by your sides, elbows soft. Drop your shoulders, then inhale and contract your abdominals.

❷ Exhale, drop your head forward and start rolling down through the spine, aiming the top of your head down to the floor and keeping your legs straight (but your knees soft).

❸ Keeping the abdominals contracted and your tailbone dropped, inhale as you roll slowly back up through the spine, vertebra by vertebra, starting at the base of the spine, bringing your head up last. Repeat 3–5 times.

❹ If your hamstrings are tight, keep your knees bent until your flexibility has increased. Focus on rolling down through the spine using a smooth, flowing movement and on keeping the abdominals contracted to support the lower back and intensify the stretch through the spine.

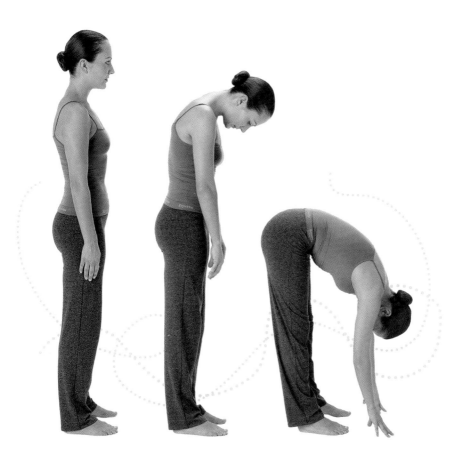

34 Neck pull prone

❶ Lie on your back in neutral with your legs extended, fingertips behind your ears and your elbows pointing out to the sides. Drop your shoulders and "soften" the chest.

❷ Inhale, contract your abdominals and exhale, raising your head and curling slowly up through the spine, one vertebra at a time. Raise up as far as you can then inhale, contract your abdominals, exhale, and roll back down. Repeat 5–10 times, lengthening out through the spine and neck as you raise and lower.

Variation—advanced

When you have developed sufficient strength in the abdominal core and flexibility in the spine, keep rolling up until you reach sitting position and curl forward, keeping the movement slow and controlled.

Inhale, contract the abdominals and exhale as you release back down.

35 Water therapy

Running water is a great energizer, as well as a cleanser. Take a trip to the restroom and hold your wrists and hands under a running tap (preferably cool) for a minute or two—you will feel recharged and refreshed.

36 Dealing with energy dips

Avoid reaching for sugary snacks or caffeine-loaded drinks to keep you going—always carry some fresh fruit, or fruit bars for those times when you need a quick fix.

37 Side bend prep

❶ Position yourself on your left side with your knees bent and your feet, ankles, and knees together. Place your left forearm on the floor, with your elbow directly beneath your left shoulder, to give you support. Lengthen through the spine as you lift the waist and ribs. Inhale.

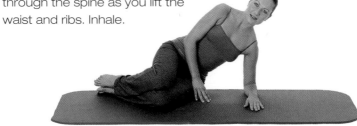

❷ Contract the abdominals and exhale, raising your hips away from the floor, keeping your knees and ankles squeezed together. Repeat 5–10 times. Change position and repeat for the other side.

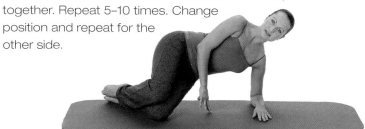

Variation—intermediate/advanced
When you are able to control this move you are ready to add in some arm movement and increase the difficulty of this exercise. As you start to raise your hips away from the floor (Step 2), curve the top arm upward in an arc, taking it over the head and creating a stretch along the right side of the body. Inhale, release the arm back down, then lower the hips. Repeat 5–10 times.

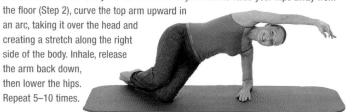

38 Chair pecs stretch

❶ Kneel on the floor with your forearm resting along the seat of a chair, your elbow at a right angle, upper arm in line with the shoulders. Inhale.

❷ Contract the abdominals, exhale, turn the head to the left, and drop the right shoulder down toward the floor. Inhale and raise. Repeat 5 times, then switch position and repeat for the other side.

39 Wrist circles

If you spend long periods at a computer keyboard, a quick way of letting go of tension in your wrists and hands and getting your energy flowing is to spend a minute or two circling your wrists, stretching your fingers as you do so.

40 Rolling back

❶ Sit with your knees raised, your legs together, hands by your hips. Inhale.

❷ Contract the abdominals, exhale and roll back, tucking your chin into your chest and using your hands to help yourself balance.

❸ Inhale and roll back up to sitting. Repeat 5–10 times, keeping the movement as smooth as possible.

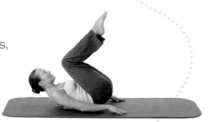

41 The hundred

Lie on the floor with your spine in neutral. Float your right leg up until your knee is at a right angle, shin parallel to the floor. Inhale, contract your abdominals, then exhale, drop your shoulders, and lengthen your arms, raising them a little. Lift and lower your arms, "pulsing" them in time with the breath: exhale for 5 pulses, then inhale for 5, until you reach 50. Change legs and repeat for the other side.

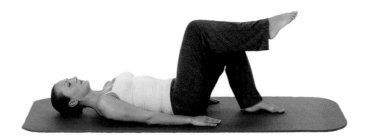

Variation—beginner/intermediate

To work the abdominal core a little harder, extend the
raised leg. The more you lower the leg, the harder you
will work the abdominals.

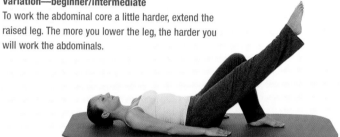

Once you have good abdominal control, try raising both legs,
first with knees bent, and then with legs extended. By now
you will be ready to keep pulsing for a count of 100.

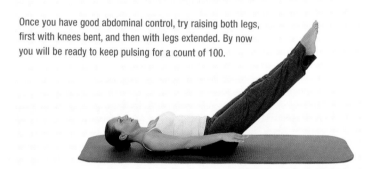

42 One o'clock jump

Never skip lunch—a proper break in the middle of the day is an important aspect in keeping yourself on top form. It not only gives you the opportunity to eat something nourishing, but also to get active and shake off any residual stress from the morning's activities. A few minutes spent carrying out some invigorating stretches will recharge and refocus your energy, enabling you to sail through the afternoon.

43 Go walkabout

Any routine that requires you to sit for long periods will result in neck and shoulder tension, and stiffness in the lower back, hips, and legs. Regularly getting up and walking around will loosen stiff muscles and get your energy flowing again.

44 Chest stretch

❶ Stand with your feet in parallel, hip-width apart. Hold a rolled-up towel or exercise band, placing your hands approximately two feet (60cm) apart. Inhale, lengthen up through the spine and neck and drop your shoulders, drawing your shoulder blades down and back.

❷ Contract the abdominals and exhale as you raise your arms up in front of you, up and over your head, and back behind you, keeping your shoulders dropped throughout. Inhale and reverse the movement, bringing your arms over and back to the starting position. Repeat 10 times, exhaling as you curve the arms back and inhaling as you return to center.

45 Shoulder bridge

❶ Lie with your spine in neutral, your arms by your sides.
Inhale. Contract the abdominals then exhale, peeling the
tailbone away from the floor very slightly.
Inhale and release back down to
the floor.

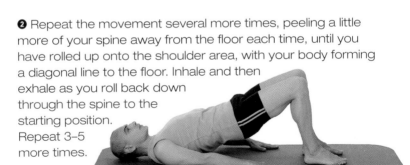

❷ Repeat the movement several more times, peeling a little
more of your spine away from the floor each time, until you
have rolled up onto the shoulder area, with your body forming
a diagonal line to the floor. Inhale and then
exhale as you roll back down
through the spine to the
starting position.
Repeat 3–5
more times.

Variation—intermediate

Once you have mastered the first part of this exercise, intensify it by adding in some arm movement. As you roll up into the diagonal position, raise your arms up and over your head. Inhale, then exhale and roll back down through the spine, leaving your arms extended behind your head. Finally, inhale and bring your arms back to the starting position. Repeat 10 times.

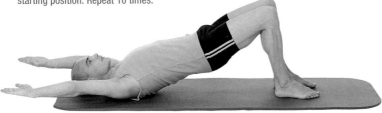

46 Flower power

Living plants and flowers have an energy that can invigorate us—keep a few fresh flowers in a vase on your desk, or table, to perk you up and raise your spirits.

47 Double leg stretch

❶ Lie on your back with your knees raised toward your chest, feet together, hands resting on the outside of your shins. Inhale and lengthen along the spine and neck.

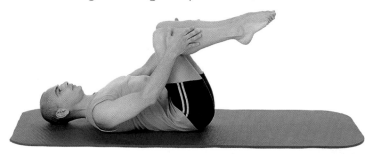

❷ Contract the abdominals and exhale as you extend your legs and slowly open your arms out to the sides. Aim to keep your legs at a forty-five-degree angle to the floor—if you are unable to keep abdominal control, raise them higher toward the ceiling.

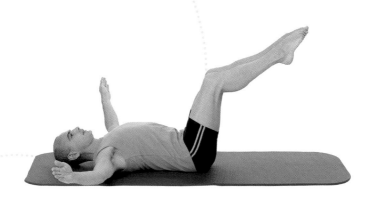

❸ Continue the movement, circling the arms round and up behind your head. Keep your shoulders dropped, your abdominals contracted and avoid arching your lower back as you extend the limbs. As you circle your arms up to the ceiling and back to the starting position, draw your knees back into your chest. Repeat 5–10 times, then 5–10 times circling the arms in the reverse direction.

48 Restoring vitality

Your immediate surroundings can do a great deal to rejuvenate or deplete your energy—try to create a clear, organized space in which to function. If you feel yourself flagging or unable to focus, take a moment to make things tidy and neat. Getting rid of any clutter or rubbish will do wonders for your energy levels.

49 Give yourself a jumpstart

Jumping up and down is a fantastic way to perk up your system, get your energy flowing, and make your spirits soar, and, best of all, it need only take a minute or two. Whenever your energy starts to flag or you're finding it hard to stay motivated, a few energizing jumps will get you back on course. Alternatively, get hold of a jumprope and do a few minutes' skipping every day to get your circulation going and help keep you physically on top form. Go on, go crazy and just jump for joy!

50 Swan dive

❶ Lie on your front with your legs extended, feet slightly apart, toes pointed. If they are uncomfortable in this position then bring your big toes in so that they are touching and drop your heels out to the sides. Place your hands just in front of your shoulders. Inhale and lengthen along the spine and neck.

❷ Contract the abdominals and inhale, lengthening up through the chest and lifting the upper body. Lift as far as is comfortable, lengthening the spine to avoid causing pressure to the lower back. Inhale and lower.
Repeat 5–10 times.

51 Spine stretch

❶ Sit with your legs positioned slightly apart, your shoulders dropped, your arms relaxed and your spine and neck lengthened. Inhale.

❷ Contract the abdominals and exhale, curving forward, as if lifting up and over a large beach ball, reaching your hands toward your feet. Inhale and curl slowly back up to center. Repeat 5–10 times.

52 Raise a smile

Give someone a friendly smile—you will raise their spirits and feel your own energy levels soar. You needn't limit yourself to the people around you either: get into the habit of answering the phone with a smile too—the person at the other end of the line may not be able to see your smile, but they will certainly be able to pick it up and feel lifted by it.

53 Leg pull (prone)

❶ Position yourself on your front then raise yourself up so that you are supporting yourself on your forearms and knees.

❷ Straighten your arms and knees, pushing yourself away from the floor, keeping your spine lengthened and your elbows soft. Inhale.

❸ Contract the abdominals and exhale, extending your left leg and raising it slightly, keeping your hips level. Inhale and lower. Repeat 5–10 times, exhaling as you raise and inhaling as you lower. Repeat for the right leg.

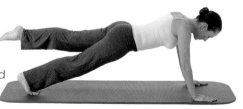

va va voom > getting physical 63

54 The side kick

❶ Lie on your left side with your legs together and your left arm extended to support your head. Rest your right hand on the floor in front of your chest, in order to help you balance.

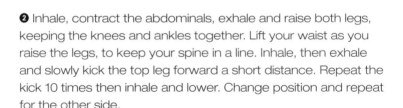

❷ Inhale, contract the abdominals, exhale and raise both legs, keeping the knees and ankles together. Lift your waist as you raise the legs, to keep your spine in a line. Inhale, then exhale and slowly kick the top leg forward a short distance. Repeat the kick 10 times then inhale and lower. Change position and repeat for the other side.

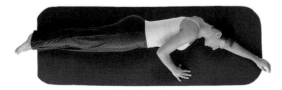

Variation—intermediate

For a more challenging version, rest the top arm along the side of your body. If you are unable to keep your balance, return the arm to its original position.

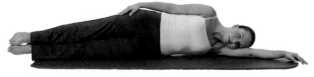

55 No matter what, no matter where

Wherever you are, whatever you're doing, use some "breathing and stretching" to let go of tension and revive you—take a couple of deep breaths—in through your nose and out through your mouth; hunch and drop your shoulders; circle your shoulders a few times in each direction; yawn widely and stretch both your arms and your legs (circumstances permitting).

56 Swimming

❶ Lie with your forehead resting on your hands. Drop your shoulders and lengthen the spine. Inhale, contract the abdominals and extend the right leg, allowing it to lift, keeping the hip in contact with the floor. Inhale and release. Repeat for the other leg. Repeat 10 times on each leg.

❷ Now work the legs in the same way but extend the left arm as you lengthen the right leg and the right arm as you lengthen the left leg. Repeat 10 times on each side.

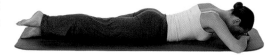

Variation—intermediate
Perform the same movement starting from a kneeling position. Keep your abdominals contracted, your hips level and the extended leg parallel to the body (avoid swinging it out to the side).

57 Take your time

No matter how busy your schedule is, take your time and avoid rushing. Hurrying to get everything done will only exhaust you and will probably result in you making unnecessary mistakes. Take a deep breath and take things at your own pace, that way you'll get them done more thoroughly (and probably more quickly than if you rush, too) and you'll be left with energy to spare.

58 Taming tension

Feeling overwhelmed and under pressure can take its toll on your physical well-being and leave you feeling jaded and weary. Soaking in a warm bath with a little lavender and rose oil will soothe tired muscles, and leave you feeling revitalized.

59 The roll up

❶ Sit upright, with your knees raised and your feet in parallel. Drop your shoulders and relax your arms. Grasp the backs of the thighs with your hands.

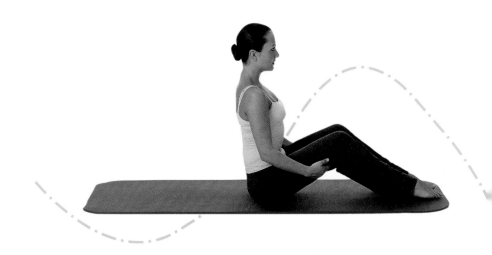

❷ Inhale, contract the abdominals and exhale as you curl back through the spine, starting at the tailbone, holding your thighs for support. When you start to feel resistance, inhale and slowly roll back up to center. Repeat 5–10 times, trying to curl back a little further each time.

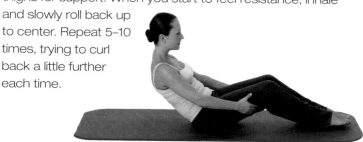

❸ Continue the move, taking your arms up and over your head, keeping your shoulders dropped. Inhale, contract the abdominals and roll slowly back up to center. Repeat the sequence 10 times.

60 Double leg kick

Lie on your front with your legs extended and your knees slightly apart. Clasp your hands behind you, drop your shoulders and lengthen through the spine and neck. Inhale then contract your abdominals. Exhale as you flick your feet toward the buttocks 3 times, squeezing your inner thighs together as you do so. Inhale and release the legs back down. Repeat 10 times.

Variation—intermediate/advanced
To intensify this exercise and increase its strengthening effect, lengthen out through the chest, raising the upper body away from the floor and focus on extending the legs even further, allowing the thighs to lift away from the floor. Repeat the flicking motion as for the variation, above. Repeat the sequence 5–10 times.

61 Reviving face massage

A five-minute massage to your face, neck, and shoulders will relax and revive you at any time of day. Rest your elbows at table height and, using the thumbs, press all the way around the eye sockets, along the cheek bones, and out to the jaw hinge. Next massage your temples with your fingertips, making little circular movements, then, still using your fingertips, gently massage the rest of your face, neck, and shoulders.

62 Let music be the food of...

If you have a personal music player, recharge your energy by sitting quietly with your eyes closed and listening to a little of your favorite music. Make sure you are sitting comfortably and take a few deep breaths. Drop your shoulders, relax your neck, and focus on letting any tension that you are holding in your body simply float away. Alternatively, put on some uplifting music and do a few energizing stretches.

63 Corkscrew

❶ Lie on your back with your legs extended, toes softly pointed and your arms by your sides, palms down.

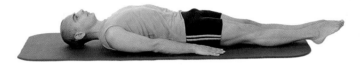

❷ Inhale, contract the abdominals and exhale, raising your legs, and lengthening along the back and neck. You can use your hands to support you.

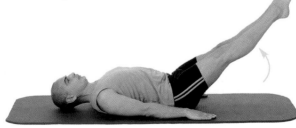

❸ Continuing to exhale as you take your legs over to the left, drawing a figure-of-eight, as you circling them down, around and up, then across to the right, circling down, around and up, and back to center.
Repeat this corkscrew motion 5–10 times. Inhale and release the legs slowly back to center.

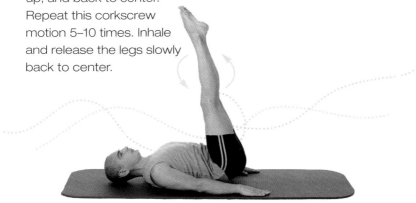

If you experience any discomfort in the lower back or difficulty in maintaining the abdominal contraction, raise your legs, taking them up to an angle of 90°, if necessary. Once your core strength and muscle control have improved, you will be able to lower your legs once more.

64 Roll over

❶ Lie on your back with your legs extended, toes softly pointed, arms by your sides, palms down.

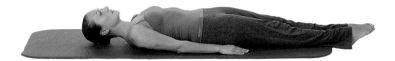

❷ Inhale, contract the abdominals and exhale as you raise your legs upward, keeping your spine in contact with the floor.

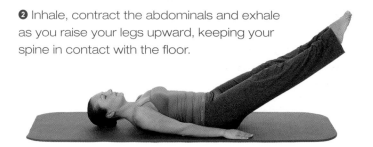

❸ Continue lifting the legs, taking your feet over your head and down toward the floor. Let your spine peel slowly away from the floor, using your hands to stabilize you, if necessary, and squeezing the buttocks as you lift.

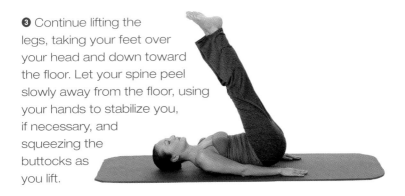

❹ When you have reached as far as you can, inhale, then exhale and roll back down through the spine, controlling the move with the abdominals. Repeat 5–10 times, increasing the stretch a little more each time.

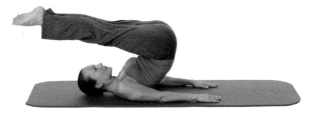

65 Winding down and letting go

At the end of a busy day spend a few minutes lying on your back with your knees bent. Breathe deeply and let any stressful thoughts float away. Now let your attention travel down through your body, starting with your head and working right down to your feet. Focus on any knots of tension and imagine breathing into them, allowing the tension to simply vanish. You will be left feeling calm and energized and ready to enjoy the evening ahead.

66 Superjuice

A glass of freshly-squeezed juice is a delicious way of recharging the body and restoring a feeling of well-being. Indulge in a refreshing glass of carrot juice—packed with minerals and vitamins (B, C, D, E, K, and beta-carotene) and excellent for improving vitality as well as calming the nerves and taking the edge off tension.

67 One leg stretch

❶ Lie on the floor with knees raised. Inhale, contract the abdominals, then exhale and extend the left leg away from you along the ground, keeping your hips level. Inhale and bring the leg back to center. Repeat 10–20 times using alternate legs.

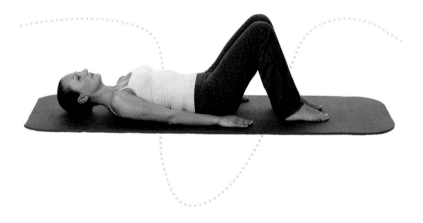

❷ Working both legs together, bring the knee up as you extend the right leg, then bring the right knee up and extend the left leg. Continue the movement, alternating the breathing and the hand position (see below) as you move the legs. Repeat for a total of 10–20 stretches.

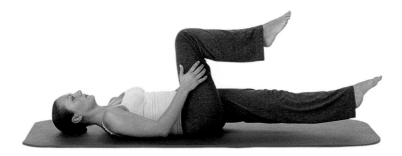

68 Hip flex

❶ Begin in a crouched position, balancing on your toes, hands on the floor either side of your feet. Slide your right leg straight back behind you, resting your right knee on the floor.

❷ Inhale, contract your abdominals then exhale as you lengthen your body forward, creating a stretch through the back of the left thigh, across the pelvis and along the front of the right thigh. Hold the stretch for 5 breaths then release. Repeat the sequence for the other side.

Variation—intermediate

For a more intense stretch, tuck the toes of your extended leg under and straighten the knee. As you exhale and lengthen forward, press the heel of the back foot down toward the floor. To further increase the stretch, rest your hands on your front knee.

69 Complete your tasks and finish your actions

Having unfinished business (however insignificant) hanging over us can be very draining, while completing tasks gives us an immediate lift. Practice completing every action that you begin, instead of putting them aside to deal with later. Start small—wash your cup as soon as you've finished with it, or return that phone call immediately.

70 Quiet time

One of the best-kept secrets for improving your vitality is to give yourself a quiet time each day to simply sit and take stock of the day and/or your state of mind and then simply let go of any worries that have been bothering you. You will be amazed at the effect that regular practise of this simple exercise can have on your feelings of well-being.

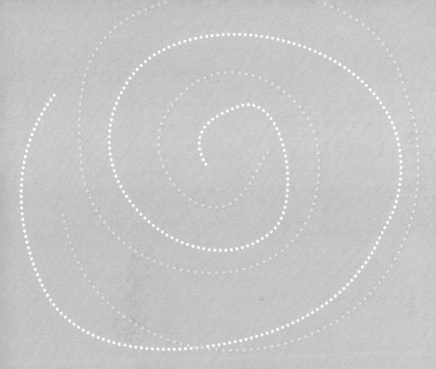

Matters of
the mind

Keeping mentally on the ball.

71 Getting ahead

Crossing the midline (the imaginary line running down through the center of the body) is a great way to boost our mental ability and get the right and left brain hemispheres working in harmony. If your mental energy suddenly fails you, or you feel unable to focus, try "cross-crawling" to get yourself back on form. Raise your left knee up and across your body, bringing your right elbow in to meet it. Release and do the same with the right knee and left elbow. Repeat this "crawling" motion for 20–30 seconds.

72 Arm circles

Stand with your feet in parallel, your left hand on your ribcage to monitor your breathing and, as you inhale, circle your right arm, raising it up over your head, then down and back round to the starting point. Repeat 5–10 times, then switch and repeat for the other arm.

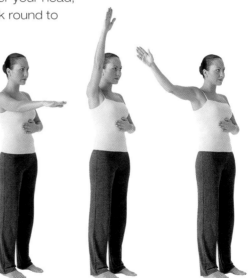

73 The saw

Sit with your legs extended, feet apart. Drop your shoulders and raise your arms, taking your left arm in front and your right arm behind. Inhale, contract the abdominals and exhale, reaching your left arm over toward your right foot. Inhale and return to center, change arms, and repeat the stretch on the other side. Repeat the sequence 5–10 times.

74 Habit forming

For exercise to have any real effect on our overall vitality we need to let it become a habit, making it as much a part of our daily routine as cleaning our teeth. Only your ongoing commitment to a regular routine of exercise, healthy eating, and adequate rest will bring about permanent, positive changes to your levels of fitness, vitality, and general well-being.

75 Climb tree

❶ Lie on your back with your legs extended. Raise the right leg and grasp the thigh with both hands.

❷ Inhale, then contract the abdominals, exhale and roll up through the spine, walking the hands up the raised leg toward the ankle in a climbing motion, lengthening the right leg away from you and lowering it slightly as you roll the body up to a sitting position. Inhale as you reverse the movement and roll back down. Repeat 5–10 times.

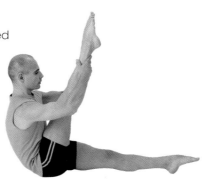

76 Spine twist

Sit with your legs extended and set as far apart as is comfortable. Raise your arms out to the sides, keeping your spine lengthened and your shoulders dropped. Inhale, contract the abdominals and exhale, rotating your upper body around to the right. Inhale and release back to center then exhale as you rotate around to the left. Repeat the sequence 10 times, increasing the stretch a little more each time.

Variation—beginner/intermediate

If the arm or leg position is uncomfortable for you, try these options instead. Position the arms either with the forearms resting one on top of the other, palms down, or in front of your chest with your fingertips touching. The legs can be either crossed at the ankles, or the soles of the feet placed together, with the knees dropped out to the sides.

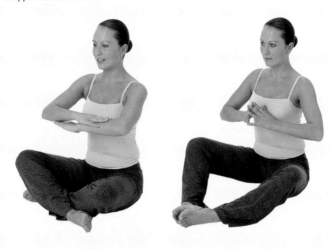

77 Open leg rocker

❶ Sit on the floor with your hands holding your ankles, toes lifted away from the floor, knees slightly apart.

❷ Inhale, contract the abdominals and, maintaining your balance, extend your left leg upward as you exhale. Inhale and release the left leg, exhale and extend the right leg. Repeat 10 times with each leg.

Variation—advanced

Extend both legs, contract the abdominals and exhale, tilting the pelvis forward as you rock slowly down through the spine. Rock as far as you can, then return to center, controlling the move with the abdominals.

78 Work soft, not hard

Changing your attitude to the way you work can have an immediate effect on your energy levels. Instead of trying to work hard all the time, why not think of working soft? When working "hard" we tense our bodies and constrict our breathing, leaving us feeling depleted and exhausted. Working soft, on the other hand, allows us to relax into the task at hand and breathe, calming the mind and attuning us to our environment, resulting in increased efficiency as well as greater vitality.

79 Positive visualization

Give yourself permission to become a healthier, happier, more vibrant you. Take a moment every day to visualize yourself as healthy, happy, and overflowing with energy. As you exercise, focus on the positive changes that are occurring to your physical and mental well-being.

80 Mental pick-me-up

A great way to give yourself a lift and release mental energy is to make yourself a to-do list. Put everything onto the list that you can think of, then examine it and decide which item is the "worst," the one that you want to avoid the most. Do that one first! You won't believe what a sense of achievement it will give you and how invigorated you will feel as a result!

81 Go easy on yourself

Learn to listen to your own body and avoid pushing yourself too far as you exercise. Taking small steps will ultimately produce much greater results, allowing you to gradually build your stamina and vitality, rather than burn yourself out. In Pilates it is much better for you to work at a lower level for longer, focusing on doing the exercises well, using the breathing and keeping the correct alignment, than to attempt a level that is actually too difficult for you.

82 Double arm stretch

❶ Lie on the floor with your spine in neutral and your knees raised. Drop your shoulders down as you inhale and slowly raise your arms up toward the ceiling.

❷ Contract the abdominals and exhale, lengthening the arms out from the shoulder sockets as you make small circles with the arms—10 circles outward and 10 inward, with the arms mirroring each other. Keep the shoulders dropped and the movements smooth.

Variation—beginner/intermediate

To work the abdominals a little harder, float the right leg up, so that the shin is parallel to the floor, and, maintaining the abdominal contraction, circle the arms 5 times in each direction, then lower the leg and repeat for the other leg.

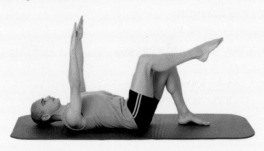

83 Exercise with a friend

Having the support of a friend can be a great way to give yourself a boost and improve your focus and concentration. Find a friend who's willing, and arrange a regular session for the two of you to exercise together.

84 Scissors

❶ Lie on your back and float your right knee up to the ceiling so that your shin is parallel to the floor. Inhale.

❷ Contract the abdominals and exhale, lowering your right foot down, as if dipping your toes into an imaginary pool of water. Repeat 5–10 times, exhaling as you dip the foot and inhaling as you raise it. Repeat for the other side. Next float both knees up, one after the other, and repeat the exercise, alternating the legs as you dip.

Variation—intermediate/advanced

Working both legs at the same time, contract the abdominals, raising and lowering the extended legs alternately in a scissoring motion, without letting them touch the floor. As you do so, rest your hands on each raised thigh in turn. Repeat for a total of 20 stretches, then inhale and release.

85 Teaser

❶ Sit with your legs extended and your arms at shoulder height. Inhale and lengthen the spine, contract the abdominals and raise your legs, squeezing your inner thighs together and leaning back to find your point of balance.

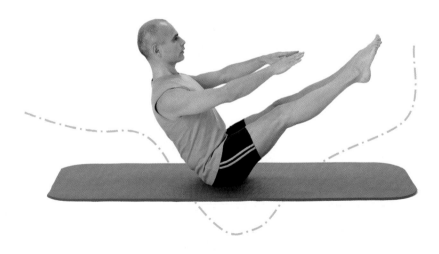

❷ Exhale and roll down through the spine, keeping your legs raised and controlling the movement with your abdominals. Inhale and roll back up, again without adjusting the legs. Repeat 5–10 times.

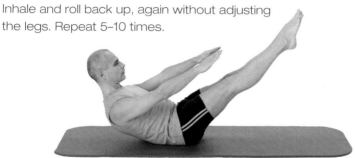

**Variation—
intermediate**
If the above position is too challenging for you, keep one foot flat on the floor until your abdominal strength improves.

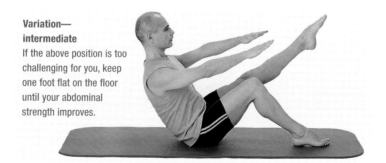

86 Side raises

❶ Lie on your left side with your head resting on your arm. Rest your right arm along your side or place your hand on the floor in front of you for support. Inhale.

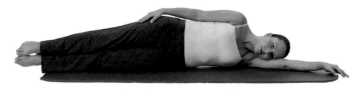

❷ Contract your abdominals and exhale, lengthening and raising the legs, squeezing the inner thighs. Keep your hips parallel, and your waist lifted. Inhale and lower. Repeat 5–10 times, then change position and repeat for the other side.

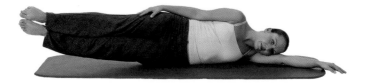

87 The crab

❶ Sit on the floor with your feet crossed and your hands supporting the ankles. Inhale, lengthen the spine, raise your feet and balancing on your sitting bones.

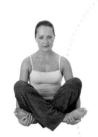

❷ Contract your abdominals, exhale and slowly roll back through your spine, vertebra by vertebra, keeping your ankles neatly tucked in and your spine curved.

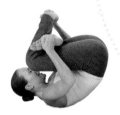

❸ Inhale, use the momentum and your abdominal muscles to help roll back up to sitting, keeping your feet raised. Repeat 5–10 times.

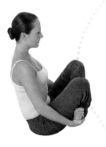

va va voom > matters of the mind 97

88 Cancan

❶ Sit with your knees bent, feet together, toes on the floor. Place your hands to either side, fingertips resting on the floor. Inhale, lengthening along the spine and neck.

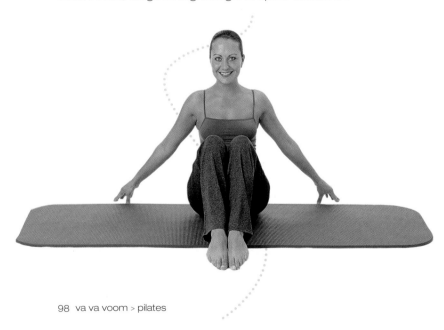

❷ Pressing your inner thighs together, contract the abdominals, exhale, and lower your knees over to the left, keeping your buttocks in contact with the floor. Inhale and bring your legs back to center, exhale and take them over to the right. Repeat this 10 times.

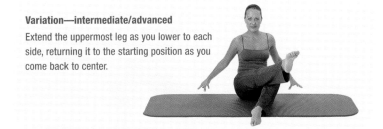

Variation—intermediate/advanced

Extend the uppermost leg as you lower to each side, returning it to the starting position as you come back to center.

89 Side kick (kneeling)

❶ Kneel with your legs slightly apart. Place your left hand on the floor directly below your left shoulder and rest the fingertips of your right hand just behind your right ear. Inhale, contract the abdominals, then exhale and extend your right leg out to the side, in line with your body allowing it to float upward away from the floor.

❷ Inhale, then exhale and move your right leg forward, without lowering it. Inhale as you take the leg back to center. Repeat 5–10 times, then change positions and repeat for the other leg.

90 Decision making

Having unresolved issues hanging over you can be very draining.
To help you find your answer and move on, try making two lists—
one showing the positive aspects and one the negative—the
outcome should then be clear. If it isn't, then maybe you're not
ready to make a decision, so, put the issue aside and forget about
it, giving yourself a time or date to come back to it. At that time,
draw up a new list and see how this compares to the old one.

91 Time management

Reaching the end of the day and wondering where the time
has gone can leave you feeling jaded: becoming aware of
exactly how you spend your time can work wonders for your
vitality levels. For one entire week list everything you do and
how long it takes. Be specific—if you're working on different
projects or activities make a note of them all. You may be
surprised at how you spend your time, but you will certainly
get a buzz from recognizing everything that you have achieved.
Once you get into the habit of writing everything down, you
will find that you become more efficient, and focused.

92 Dealing with stress

When you're feeling stressed, or overwhelmed and unable to think clearly, it can be tempting to either retreat into yourself or simply allow whatever is worrying you to dominate your thoughts, draining you mentally and emotionally. Taking some deep breaths and doing a few stretches will help you to feel balanced in mind and body, giving you a renewed sense of perspective and leaving you feeling refreshed and able to cope with the pressures that were previously weighing you down.

93 Glute stretch

❶ Lie on your back with your legs raised, knees bent. Cross your left ankle over your right knee and place your hands around your right thigh.

❷ Contract your navel in toward your spine and exhale as you gently pull your right thigh into your chest, creating a stretch in the left leg. Repeat 5 times, breathing in through the nose and out through the mouth, trying to increase the stretch each time. Inhale and release. Repeat for the other side.

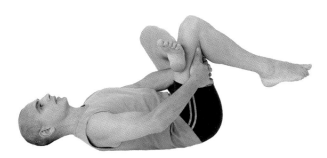

94 Plank

❶ Lie face down with your elbows in line with your shoulders and your forearms resting on the floor, hands palms downward. Drop your shoulders. Inhale.

❷ Contract the abdominals, exhale, and raise yourself up slowly onto your knees keeping the spine and neck lengthened and the shoulders dropped.

❸ Inhale and tuck your toes under, then exhale and slowly straighten your legs, pushing your knees away from the ground. Keep controlling the move with the abdominals and make sure the body is in a line, parallel to the floor. Inhale in this position then exhale as you lower gently back down onto your knees. Repeat 5–10 times.

95 Revitalizing aromas

Nice smells can raise your spirits, calm your mind and clarify your thinking. There are many essential oils to choose from: try some lavender, bergamot, lemon or rose. If you can, get hold of an oil burner, otherwise sprinkle a few drops of oil on a tissue and keep it close at hand.

96 Staying in the flow

Adopt a positive attitude to life—you'll find that people brimming over with vitality and zest for life tend to be naturally optimistic and enthusiastic. Remember, 85 per cent of the negative things that we worry about never actually happen—so why waste energy worrying about them?

97 The seal

❶ Sit on the floor with your knees and ankles together, your hands resting on your shins. Now raise your feet off the ground and lean back very slightly to find your point of balance. Hold this position as you inhale and lengthen up along the spine.

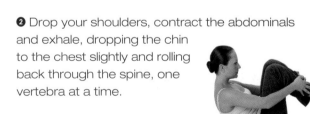

❷ Drop your shoulders, contract the abdominals and exhale, dropping the chin to the chest slightly and rolling back through the spine, one vertebra at a time.

❸ When you have rolled back as far as possible, clap your feet together 3 times (like a seal), inhale and roll slowly back up to center. Repeat 5–10 times.

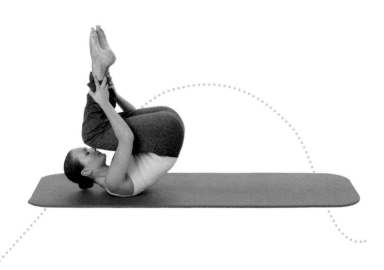

98 Cat

❶ Kneel on all fours with your knees beneath your hips and your hands beneath your shoulders, arms straight. Inhale and lengthen along the spine.

❷ Contract your abdominals, drop your chin toward your chest, tuck your pelvis under and, using a slow, smooth movement, arch your back up toward the ceiling as you exhale. Inhale and release back to the starting position.

❸ Exhale and lift your tailbone and head upward while curving your body down toward the floor. Inhale and release. Repeat the sequence 5–10 times.

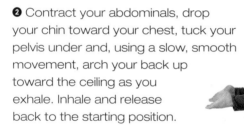